DEMENTIA

NO STIGMA OR STEREOTYPE REQUIRED

BEULAH SHADRACHE

DEMENTIA:

NO STIGMA OR STEREOTYPE REQUIRED

Published by Beulah Shadrache Consultants Ltd.

The Green, Datchet, Berkshire, SL3 9AS

ISBN: 978-0-7961-2903-1

Cover image by Michael Dayce

Images by Michael Dayce

Dedication

I dedicate this book to every person who has a diagnosis of dementia and to every family member, neighbour, social worker, caregiver, therapist, doctor, neurologist and any other allied health and social care professional who is involved in their care and support.

Together, we can educate and empower others to understand dementia and reduce the stigma and stereotypes associated with it.

I stand with you.

Beulah Shadrache

Acknowledgment

I wish to express my gratitude to the following people who have been instrumental in making the publication of this book a reality: to my mum, Johanna Dayce, with whom I share my first memories of sitting at the dining room table writing essays; to Beryl Small, administrator for enABLE Foundation, for her diligence in sacrificing her time to proofread the manuscript of this book; and to my best friend and dear husband, Rodgell Shadrache, for his unwavering love and support.

Above all, I thank God for the gifts, talents and abilities He has endowed me with. I choose to use these to advance His kingdom on earth as I support those whose lives are impacted by dementia.

Beulah

CONTENT

FOREWORD

Stigma plays a major role in how people with dementia are perceived and treated in society. Unsympathetic labels and flawed beliefs about dementia cause people with dementia to be stereotyped, stigmatised, and marginalised.

The aim of writing this book is to help create dementia-friendly communities. I do not believe that enough people have adequate knowledge and understanding of dementia to empathise with and support people with dementia. I trust that by reading this book it will, at least, give the reader a clearer understanding of dementia which, in turn, will develop greater empathy towards those living with dementia.

I am sure that as you pick up this book you would already have heard the word 'dementia'. Now my question is: In your own words, can you explain to someone what dementia is? If you are thinking that you will say that it is 'a disease that causes old people to forget things', then I would like to invite you to carry on reading.

INTRODUCTION

Before we dive into the topic of dementia, I want to invite you to pause and spend time thinking about some of the people whom you've had in your life up to this point. If you choose, you can take out pen and paper and write down the names of individuals. Your list can include whom you choose but can range from your parents, siblings, children, grandchildren, parents-in-law, bothers-and-sisters-in-law, nephews, nieces to neighbours, friends, colleagues, and acquaintances. Now focus on each person in turn, thinking about their physical appearances, personalities, the work they do or subjects they are good at, their talents, and hobbies. Is the person sporty, intellectually gifted, artistic, or creative? Then consider their temperaments; is the person gentle, soft-spoken, funny, jovial, energetic, sad, or negative? Does the person enjoy socialising? What do they prefer: the company of close family and friends or going out with friends and making new ones?

I am sure that for each person you would be able to provide information for most, if not all, of the above. Every person is unique in their own way, be it in their physical appearance, temperaments, abilities, and preferences. No two people are the same, even if they are identical twins! And this is the most important fact to remember when it comes to dementia. We will look at what dementia is in the first chapter, but there is one thing that dementia is not...the person! So, I want you to hold onto this nugget of truth as you continue to read this book. Too often, dementia is allowed to rob an individual of their personhood - being a human being with distinguishing characteristics, likes, dislikes, abilities, strength, weaknesses, opinions, preferences, dreams, and the list goes on.

If we are going to make a difference in how people with dementia are seen and treated, then we have to start with the person. We must recognise that before someone's diagnosis of dementia, s/he was able to give expression to who they are, and, if given the opportunity and time to do so - and not be tarnished with the dementia-stereotypes brush - will still be able to do so. We need to focus on the person and not the dementia.

A trend that has taken social media by storm is people posting pictures of their loved ones who have dementia. Sadly, many images are of those at the end of life. When one looks at social media feeds you will find that daily there are several posts of people with dementia... without their permission! People just take liberties to post: mums, dads, grandmothers, grandfathers, uncles, aunts, and even service users have become nothing more than a picture depicting dementia. This is shocking, unacceptable, and a horrendous violation of the individual's personhood. How this makes sense to anyone boggles the mind. No one posts pictures of loved ones with heart disease, kidney failure, lung cancer, etc. Yet, as is the case with all these medical conditions, dementia is simply a condition that involves a disorder of a body organ - the brain - and not some out-of-space phenomenon that requires those with the condition to be spread across social media platforms as if they have become some universal commodity that the public has the right to be entertained with. Added to this, unhelpful references to people with dementia as 'suffers' reinforces a negative narrative in which individuals with dementia are undermined, dehumanised, and in some cultures, even demonised - especially women - and referred as witches. No one refers to someone with diabetes, cardiovascular disease or asthma as sufferers, so why do it to people with dementia? The answer: a lack of understanding of the condition.

Every person who has dementia has the right to be treated as a person - a human being. The minute we lose sight of this, we have lost the fight against dementia. Once we understand and appreciate this, we are well on our way to winning the battle against dementia. Each one of us has a responsibility to decide whether we want to be part of the problem or the solution; whether to continue posting images and reinforcing negative perceptions of people with dementia or to stop doing so and become an advocate who speaks and acts against this vile practice. Those who choose to continue this demeaning practice need to consider whether they would be happy for others to do the same should they develop the condition.

My challenge to you

Before you start reading the first chapter, I would like to challenge you to look towards the back of the book where you will find a quiz. You can decide how you attempt the quiz, but I would like to suggest that you complete it before you start reading and record your score as your first attempt in the table provided. Then, repeat the quiz after you've read the book. If preferred, you can attempt the quiz one chapter at a time. Approach it in whichever way will work best for you. However, your score should increase significantly after having read all the information contained in the book, which will be great, as the aim of writing the book would be achieved...to increase your knowledge and understanding of dementia.

The quiz is very easy to complete, as all you have to do is to select 'True' or 'False'. The answers follow after the test, so you will be able to check how much information you've retained. This will provide you with a good idea of any information in the book you need to revisit.

Chapter One

What is Dementia?

"Dementia is not a disease."

One of the most common errors that people make is to say that dementia a disease. I have even heard healthcare professionals make this statement. I want to emphasise that dementia is not a disease. At this point you may say: "Ok, so if dementia is not a disease, what is it?" In answer to this question and to illustrate what dementia is, I make use of what I call the fruit bowl analogy.

Please look at the picture below.

If I asked you to tell me what is in the bowl, you will answer that it is fruit. Fruit is the collective name (noun) that we use for all these different items we see in the bowl. If I asked you to name the items in the bowl, you would say there are grapes, apples, oranges, lemons, cherries, pears, etc.

Now look at the picture below.

If I asked what you see, you would tell me it is an orange.

If I've not seen an orange before and I asked you what an orange is, you would reply that it is a fruit.

Now look at the next image below. I have separated some of the fruit from the others.

We know that all these objects are called fruit and even if we separated each one of them, it will still be called a fruit. However, the fruit I have separated can be grouped together as a particular type of fruit, namely citrus fruit. When we look at the fruit in the group, we see they have different shapes, colours, and sizes. Their skin is very similar, but some are tougher than others. They have other similarities: citrus fruits are juicy and are divided into segments. However, they have differences in taste as some are sweet, some are tangy, and some are very sour!

We can now apply this analogy (illustration) to dementia. Like the word 'fruit', dementia is a collective word (noun), or we can say an umbrella term that is used for a variety of diseases such as Alzheimer's disease, vascular disease, and syndromes such as Wernicke-Korsakoff syndrome that cause damage to the brain. I will explain this in greater detail when we look at the different types of dementia (like different types of fruit), and how some cause similar and some cause different symptoms, just like the fruits have similarities and differences.

So now we know that dementia is an umbrella term or syndrome (collection of symptoms) used to describe the symptoms of different diseases and syndromes (conditions characterised by several symptoms, such as Downs Syndrome). However, as there are so many misconceptions about dementia, let us separate fact from fiction.

Some truths about dementia

- There are over 200 types of dementia.
- There are currently over 55 million people living with dementia worldwide.
- Someone develops dementia every 3 seconds.
- Every year more than 10 million people develop dementia.
- There is currently no cure for dementia.
- Dementia affects both men and women.
- Dementia is progressive, meaning that the symptoms a person will experience will increase over time.
- Dementia does affect a person's memory, thinking, behaviour, emotions, and abilities.
- People with dementia can still live a very productive life but may need support with some things.
- Dementia is not a natural part of growing old.

- Dementia does not affect everyone in the same way.
- People with dementia still have lots of abilities.
- People with dementia have their own unique experience.
- Dementia is not caused by witchcraft and women who have dementia are not witches.
- Dementia can be prevented.

Some untruths about dementia

- Dementia is an old people's disease.
- Only people over the age of 65 develop dementia.
- There is nothing that can be done when someone has dementia.
- Dementia takes over the person's identity.
- People with dementia can't remember anything.
- People with dementia are unable to do things for themselves.
- Only medication can improve symptoms of dementia.

- All people with dementia are affected in the same way, so we must treat them all the same.
- Media reports about dementia are always accurate.
- People with dementia are senile.
- People with dementia don't know or understand what's going on around them.
- People with dementia always need others to make their decisions for them.
- People with dementia are aggressive.
- People with dementia go back to being a child.

We have now not only identified exactly what dementia is but have also highlighted some of the truths and untruths about dementia. Take time to read through the above statements again, until you have a clear picture of dementia. This should have an immediate impact on the way you view and approach people living with dementia.

We will explore each statement further as we progress through the book.

Chapter Two

Causes of Dementia

'There are over 200 known causes of dementia'

Types of Dementia

When referring to the types of dementia, we refer to what causes the dementia; in other words what causes the symptoms that the person is experiencing.

We will now look at the different types of dementia. As mentioned in the first chapter, there are over 200 types, so it will not be possible to cover all of them in this book. I will, however, look at the most common types of dementia, as well as some of the less-known types.

More common types of dementia

Alzheimer's disease is the most common type of dementia, affecting around 60-70 percent of people who have dementia. A person's brain has billions of nerve cells that need to connect with one another so that messages can be passed between cells. See it as a mobile phone network with text messages, WhatsApp messages and phone calls going back and forth from one to another. Alzheimer's disease, through the build-up of proteins, causes 'plaques' and 'tangles' in the brain cells. These 'tangles' and 'plagues' prevent the signals (messages) from being passed between the cells. Over time the cells shrink, and eventually die. Also, our brains have chemicals that help pass on messages between cells. In Alzheimer's disease, people have fewer of these chemicals, meaning that messages cannot be passed on between the cells. Alzheimer's is progressive - in other words, more and more cells are affected as time goes on. Below is a diagram of a healthy brain, and one affected by Alzheimer's disease.

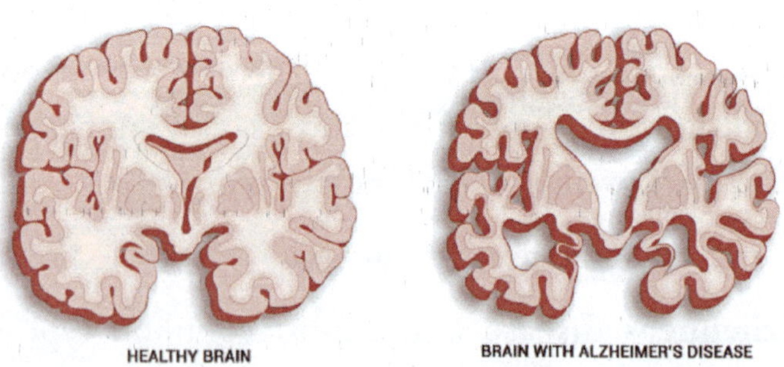

Vascular disease is the second most common type of dementia. It occurs when there is a problem with the supply of blood to the brain. Blood forms the transport system in the body that carries oxygen and nutrients to the cells, including the brain cells. When there is not enough supply of blood to the brain cells then the cells are starved of oxygen and nutrients, and eventually die. Blood supply to the brain cells can either be cut off because a blood vessel, through which the blood flows, has burst, or because there is something in the blood vessel (usually a clot) that is blocking the blood from flowing through to get to the cells.

There are several types of vascular dementia. Each type is identified by what damage it causes to the brain and where in the brain the damage takes place. Some of the symptoms of the different types of vascular dementia are similar, but some are different. (Remember the citrus fruit: similar in some features, but different in others.) How it affects people is different for each type. So, let's look at the different types.

Stroke-related dementia

When someone has a stroke, the blood supply to cells in the brain is cut off. This supply cut-off can either be temporary or permanent. It can also occur in different parts of the brain. Where it occurs and whether it is a temporary or permanent event will determine how seriously the stroke affects the person.

Post-stroke dementia

When the blood supply in one of the large blood vessels in the brain is cut off, then it causes a major stroke. This can happen because of a blood clot in the blood vessel or as a result of the blood vessel bursting, which causes bleeding into the brain. About 20 percent of people who experience such a major stroke develop post-stroke dementia. A person who has had a stroke is at risk of having more strokes and is at greater risk of developing dementia.

Single-infarct and multi-infarct dementia

These types of dementia are caused by smaller strokes that occur in medium-sized or larger blood vessels, due to a clot. Sometimes the person may not even be aware that they had a stroke, as the blockage may clear itself or the symptoms of a stroke may only last a few minutes. This is known as a mini-stroke.

Lewy Body dementia is the third most common type of dementia. It is often mistaken as Alzheimer's disease. Lewy bodies are proteins that build up in the nerve cells of the brain. It is believed that Lewy bodies form because of low levels of certain chemicals in the brain.

These chemicals are responsible for carrying messages between nerve cells. When the connection between nerve cells doesn't take place, the cells die.

Frontotemporal dementia refers to a range of different conditions. It is also called Pick's disease or frontal lobe dementia. Frontotemporal refers to two parts of the brain; the frontal lobe, which is just behind your forehead, above your eyebrows, and the temporal lobe which is on either side of your head, just above the ears.

Mixed dementia occurs when a person has more than one type of dementia, and the most common combination is Alzheimer's disease and vascular dementia. Another combination is Alzheimer's disease and Lewy body dementia.

Other types of dementia

Young-onset dementia refers to dementia that develops in people under the age of 65. It can also be referred to as early-onset dementia. Various diseases can cause young-onset dementia and often it is caused by a rarer form of dementia.

Alcohol-related brain damage (ARBD) is caused by heavy drinking over long periods of time. The most common form of ARBD is alcoholic dementia, otherwise known as alcohol-related dementia. It includes a condition called Korsakoff's syndrome.

AIDS-related cognitive impairment occurs in people affected by HIV and AIDS, especially in the later stages of their illness.

Dementia associated with **Parkinson's disease (DPD)** is understood to be caused by proteins called Lewy's bodies.

I trust this chapter has provided you with a better understanding of the different causes of dementia and that you can now appreciate how different the symptoms will be for each person. We will discuss the different symptoms in the next chapter.

Chapter Three

Symptoms of Dementia

"Forewarned is forearmed"

The more knowledge we have of a condition, the better equipped we are to identify signs and symptoms of the condition. This rings true for dementia. As discussed in the first chapter, the number of people living with dementia is on the rise, drastically and globally. Whilst there is no cure currently for dementia, we know that there are things we can do to help reduce our chances of developing dementia. Having said that, there are no guarantees that someone will not get dementia. So, we all have a responsibility to equip ourselves, not only with knowledge and understanding of how to reduce our risk of dementia, but to be informed to recognise the signs and symptoms of dementia, not only in others, but in ourselves as well. How do we do this? By being proactive and signing up for opportunities where we can get expert information on the subject. I want to share a word of caution here: be careful where you get your information from. Only allow those who have expertise in this subject to inform you. The more accurate information you gather, the more empowered you become.

So, let's look at some symptoms associated with dementia. Bear in mind that I am only providing information on some of the symptoms. In line with the previous chapter, I want to compare and contrast different types of dementia and the symptoms they present.

Symptoms associated with Alzheimer's disease

- Memory loss that disrupts daily life
- Misplacing things
- Losing track of dates
- Not remembering current location
- Taking longer to complete usual daily tasks
- Repeating questions / not remembering recently learnt information
- Finding planning or solving problems difficult

- Loss of spontaneity and sense of taking initiative
- Difficulty handling money and paying bills
- Difficult completing tasks such as personal care, e.g. bathing, oral care.
- Wandering from a familiar environment and having difficulty in finding the way back.
- Increased anxiety and agitation
- Mood and personality changes

Remember, all of us can occasionally experience the symptoms above, and more so, when we are under tremendous pressure, experiencing a trauma or feeling stressed. I can certainly hold my hand up as one who has put fresh milk in the cupboard, added sugar instead of salt to a meal, experienced times where I've not had the energy to start a new project, and not remembered where I parked my car when exiting a shopping centre. And I'm sure you can too. My children will be the first to tell you that they have been called by their sibling's name. Not any of these experiences indicated that I had dementia and neither do yours. However, when there is a pattern of symptoms which increase in frequency then it is time to have it checked out.

Symptoms asociated with Dementia with Lewy Bodies (DLB)

Dementia with Lewy bodies refer to two related diagnoses - Lewy body dementia (LBD) and Parkinson's disease dementia (PDD). Symptoms include:

- Muscle rigidity or stiffness
- Shuffling walk, slow movement, or frozen stance
- Tremor or shaking, most commonly at rest
- Balance problems and repeated falls
- Stooped posture
- Loss of coordination
- Smaller handwriting than was usual for the person
- Reduced facial expression
- Difficulty swallowing
- A weak voice
- Changes in alertness and attention, and periods of confusion. These periods can be unpredictable and change from hour-to-hour, or day-to-day.
- Visual hallucinations. People with DLB may see things that are not there, for example, people or animals. These hallucinations can happen

repeatedly and are realistic.

- Sleep problems. Vivid dreams and shouting out or moving while asleep. This can disrupt sleep and may cause injury.
- Changes to thinking and memory. People often notice difficulty planning activities, and loss of ability to find their way around. Memory can be affected, but this may occur later and is often less affected.
- Mood and emotions. Depression and anxiety are commonly seen in DLB but can often be alleviated with treatment.
- Changes to a sense of smell or taste.

Yet again, some of us may have experienced some of the symptoms above, but these may have been caused by other conditions or circumstances. Someone who has an ear infection, for example, or even a urinary tract infection, may appear unsteady on their feet. We may also experience difficulty swallowing when we have a throat infection or experience challenges with sleep which affect our ability to concentrate the following day and affect our mood. Yet again, I can identify totally; having eight hours of sleep works best for me.

Symptoms associated with vascular dementia

It is not unusual for symptoms of post-stroke dementia to occur immediately or soon after the person had a stroke.

Symptoms in small vessel disease are more likely to develop in a more gradual way, meaning the symptoms will get worse over time. However, how quick or slow change occurs can vary over time and is different from one person to another.

Vascular dementia symptoms may include:

- Slower thinking - taking more time to process information, follow instructions or to plan ahead.
- Speaking – struggling to find the right words, slurring speech or difficulty following conversations.
- Personality changes – people may experience low mood, not feel motivated, be more emotional, or lose interest in what's happening around them.
- Movement problems and stability - difficulty or unsteadiness walking or changes in the way a person walks.

As mentioned, symptoms get worse over time. At the advanced stage of dementia, the condition affects most aspects of the person's daily life. This means that over time someone with vascular dementia may need help and support with eating, drinking, washing, dressing, walking, and using the toilet. The individual may need aids such as crockery and cutlery designed to meet the needs of people with dementia in mind, walking aids, and many other aids to support their daily living. There is a vast range of aids available.

Symptoms associated with frontotemporal dementia (FTD)

The symptoms of frontotemporal dementia can be very different to the symptoms associated with other common forms of dementia such as Alzheimer's disease, which includes memory loss and confusion.

The early symptoms of frontotemporal dementia vary from person to person and depend on which area of the brain is affected first.

Symptoms may include:

Changes in emotions - a change in how people express their feelings or understand other people's feelings. For example, someone with FTD may not recognise when someone else is upset.

Lack of interest - becoming withdrawn or losing interest in everyday life. Someone with FTD may stop looking after him/herself. The person may refuse to have a wash, brush their teeth, or change clothing.

Inappropriate behaviour - making inappropriate jokes or behaving 'strangely' in front of others. Someone with FTD may show a change in sense of humour, or sexual behaviour may change. Some people with FTD may become impulsive or easily distracted.

Obsessions – some individuals may develop new beliefs, interests, or obsessions. A very common example is the need to shop and buying what the person does not need or buying too many of the same thing. This can happen daily, several times a day. Developing a new gambling habit is another example.

Diet – changes in food likes and dislikes such as eating lots of sweet things, over-eating or drinking too much.

Awareness – individuals may not realise that they are experiencing changes in their personality or behaviour. However, the changes can become very upsetting to family members.

Decision-making - individuals may experience difficulty making plans, following instructions, and deciding what to do.

Communication – individuals may experience difficulties with speaking and understanding words. The person may therefore repeat words and phrases, struggle to say the right word or forget what words mean.

Recognition - individuals may have difficulty recognising people or knowing what objects are for. For example, a person may not recognise that a kettle is used to boil water or that the remote controls the television.

Memory - day-to-day memory may be less affected in the early stages of FTD, but problems with attention and concentration can be common.

Movement problems - around one in every eight people with behavioural variant FTD also develops movement problems of motor neurone disease. This can include stiff or twitching muscles, muscle weakness and difficulty swallowing.

Forms of frontotemporal dementia:

Behavioural variant frontotemporal dementia - in individuals with this type of dementia, the parts of the frontal lobe (see Chapter 4) that control social behaviour may be most affected. This means changes in behaviour, emotion and awareness are the most common symptoms.

Semantic dementia - the parts of the temporal lobe that support understanding of language and factual knowledge are most affected. This means individuals forget the names of objects and can struggle with concepts, like money and paying for items.

Progressive non-fluent aphasia - the parts of the frontal lobe that control speech are most affected. This is associated with individuals struggling to find the right words or have difficulty carrying a conversation.

Frontotemporal dementia is a progressive condition. Over time symptoms get worse and an individual may need more support on a day-to-day basis, decreasing their independence, and therefore, increasing their dependence on others.

People with FTD may also experience difficulties with eating, swallowing, communication, as well as with bladder and bowel control, meaning they may become incontinent. Some individuals with FTD may also develop problems with movement like those experienced by people with Parkinson's disease.

I trust you can now appreciate how important it is to seek professional advice as soon as you or someone close to you shows symptoms which are persistent and increasing in frequency. The first step would be to request a formal assessment. We will explore this in our next chapter.

Chapter Four

Assessment for Dementia

'Without a formal diagnosis, there is no dementia'

The first step to take when you experience or see someone having symptoms of dementia, as described in the previous chapter, is to have a diagnostic assessment done. The sooner this is done, the better. The aim of a diagnostic assessment is to find out if someone has dementia or whether there are other reasons for the symptoms the person is experiencing, and, if dementia is present, what type of dementia it is. Unfortunately, too often, seeking help in this area is delayed; more than often because of the stigma attached to dementia. No one should have to fear seeking advice and support when dementia is suspected, as delaying the process would not have any benefit, but will only delay treatment and support that could improve the person's wellbeing and quality of life. This highlights the need to educate society so that individuals will not feel fearful when facing the possibility of having dementia. The sooner dementia is diagnosed, the sooner treatment can start, and the necessary support be put in place. It is very important that we do not assume that someone has dementia because they show certain characteristics; there has to be a formal diagnosis. It is of the utmost importance that the person's dignity is maintained throughout the whole process of finding out whether s/he has dementia. It is equally important for the person to remain in control of their own lives and to take a lead role in the decisions-making process (unless this is not possible) regarding the way forward.

Where to start

The first step to take when there are possible signs of dementia is to see a doctor so that a medical examination can be carried out. The doctor will check whether there is, for example, any signs of an infection in someone's waterworks. Having a urine infection can cause confusion, dizziness, and agitation. These could be misread as symptoms of dementia when the truth is that it can be treated very quickly with a course of antibiotics.

Once the doctor has ruled out any physical illnesses, then the person can be referred to a memory clinic. A memory clinic specialises in carrying out tests to see if a person has problems with their brain function, including their memory. This is therefore a place where a diagnosis of dementia can be made. If this service is not available in your area, then a referral to a neurologist is needed.

Getting a diagnosis

It is very important that different healthcare professionals are involved in the process of diagnosing dementia. A doctor, for example will be familiar with the person's medical history, as well as the factors that will put the person at risk of developing dementia. A neurologist will be able to assess how well the person's brain is functioning. A psychiatrist will address mental health challenges, such as depression and anxiety, and a psychologist may be involved in helping the person to work through some past traumas. A nurse may be involved in nursing care, such as treating diabetes, and a caregiver may help someone who is recovering from an operation or accident such as a fall. An occupational therapist may be required to make the necessary adjustments in the person's home, such as identifying whether handrails are required to aid mobility. These are only a few of the key role players who may need to be involved in the person's support and, together, they will have a common goal to achieve the best health and well-being outcomes for the individual.

Chapter Five

Medicine to Treat Dementia

'Misuse of medication is abuse'

There are two classes of medication used to treat dementia. I want to emphasise that, at this stage, there is currently no cure for dementia. The purpose of the medicine is to improve functioning and to manage symptoms. It is very important that the person with dementia, as far as possible, is involved in making a decision about the medication they will use to treat their symptoms. It is equally important that a person who lacks capacity, meaning they are not able to make decisions due to damage to the brain, is supported by someone who has their best interests at heart, and can make decisions on their behalf. Medication should never be used to control a person with dementia's behaviour and should not be given in a covert (e.g., hidden in food) way, unless this is absolutely necessary and authorised by healthcare professionals. Giving medication in an unauthorised way is a form of abuse!

Medicine usually has two names, the generic name, which tells us what it is made of and the brand name. For example, you will be very familiar with medicine called 'aspirin', which is the generic name, and you may buy it as 'Dispirin', which is the brand name.

As mentioned at the start of this chapter, there are two classes of medicine used to treat dementia. Each class of medication works differently. The first type of medicine is prescribed under three different names, namely donepezil, rivastigmine and galantamine. These are their generic names.

Donepezil is licensed as Aricept, but the generic name is more commonly used.

Rivastigmine was originally licensed as Exelon, but can also be prescribed with other brand names, as well as by its generic name.

Galantamine was originally licensed as Reminyl, but is also prescribed as generic galantamine, as well as other brand names: Reminyl XL, Acumor XL, Galsya XL and Gatalin XL.

The second class of medication prescribed for dementia was originally licensed Ebixa but is currently available as generic memantine. There are also other brand names.

The first class of medication is useful in the treatment of mild to moderate Alzheimer's disease.

Memantine is used in moderate and severe Alzheimer's disease or when the person is intolerant of the other medicines.

When prescribing any of these medicines, it is essential to consider any other medication that the person is taking to avoid severe side effects.

There are several factors to consider when prescribing medication for the different sub-types of dementia. It is therefore essential that a team of healthcare professionals are involved in the process, from diagnosis to prescribing.

How do these drugs work?

The first class of medicine called acetylcholinesterase inhibitors (generally referred to as

cholinesterase inhibitor) attaches itself to the enzyme, cholinesterase, and prevents it from breaking down the neurotransmitter, acetylcholine, which help send the messages between nerve cells. As a result, with the presence of more acetylcholine in the brain, there is better communication between the nerve cells. This may help reduce the symptoms the person experiences due to Alzheimer's disease; for example, the person may be able to communicate better.

The second class of medication used to treat dementia, memantine, decreases abnormal activity in the brain. Glutamate is a chemical in the brain that sends messages between nerve cells in the brain. Nerve cells in the brain that are damaged by Alzheimer's disease make too much glutamate which cause more damage to the brain. Memantine protects nerve cells by blocking the effects of too much glutamate. Memantine may improve the ability to think and remember or may help people who have Alzheimer's disease to maintain these abilities for longer.

Chapter Six

The Human Brain

'The brain is neuroplastic, meaning it can change'

I describe the brain as the cockpit or control tower of the body. It is the centre of the body from where all bodily functions are controlled. You can lift a spoon with your hand because the brain sends messages to the muscle cells in your arm to do so. You can walk, placing one foot in front of the other, because the brain sends messages to the cells in your legs and feet to do so. You can remember things because connections between cells in the brain enable you to do so. You know not to undress yourself in public, because there is a part in your brain that will let you know that it will not be appropriate or socially acceptable to do so. You can have a conversation with someone, forming meaningful sentences, because cells in your brain form connections to enable you to do so. You can control when you go to toilet, because the brain sends messages to your bladder to hold on to the urine, until you get to the toilet. You were able to decide what to wear today, because you were able to think about what you have in your wardrobe, consider the weather outside, know whether you are going to the beach or to work. It would not have been very appropriate if you work in an office, and you turned up in your swimwear! I think you may have been sent home straight away! You were also able to choose a matching pair of shoes this morning as you were able to see the colour, style, and design of each shoe. Here I have to come clean and admit that many years ago, as a 26-year-old secondary school teacher, I did turn up to school one day with a mismatched pair of tan shoes; the one shoe had a rubber sole and the other a wooden heel. The one had a pattern and the other was plain! The cause of my dilemma was that I had a three-month-old baby sleeping in her cot, right next to the built-in cupboard where my shoes were kept. I did not turn on the light as I did not want to wake her. My pupils and colleagues had their entertainment for the day! This drives home the fact that we cannot go by symptoms alone.

Sadly, many people with dementia are not always able to

enjoy the benefits of a brain that is serving them in a way that enables them to perform all daily living tasks, due to damage to a particular part or different parts of their brain.

At this point I just want to give a short overview of the structure of the brain, what each part of the brain is responsible for, and how damage to each area can limit the person with dementia.

The brain is made up of different parts and is divided into a forebrain, midbrain and hindbrain. The forebrain is very vulnerable to causes of dementia. The brain is also divided into a left side and a right side, or hemispheres as we call it, each having four lobes and each lobe has specific functions.

See table below with names of lobes and their functions.

Table 1.1 Four brain lobes with key functi ons		
Lobe	**Position**	**Function**
Frontal lobe	Above eyebrows	Behaviour, planning and decision -making
Parietal lobe	Top of head	Body control and space
Temporal	Above each ear	Understanding, memory, and language
Occipital	At the back of the head	Vision

Although each lobe is responsible for specific functions, it is essential for the different lobes to communicate with one another. To demonstrate, the occipital lobe is responsible for vision. However, there needs to be communication between the occipital and temporal lobes for us to make sense of what we see. It may therefore be possible that the person who has dementia is able to see well, but because there is damage to the temporal lobe, the person cannot make sense of what, or sometimes who, they see. A parent with dementia may therefore not recognise their own child.

The frontal lobe, on the other hand, takes in knowledge from the temporal and parietal lobes to enable us to make decisions about actions and behaviour. When there is a breakdown in communication between these lobes, due to damage to the brain cells, then the process cannot be completed.

Contrary to the old belief that the brain is unchangeable and wears away with age, there is now a lot of evidence to show that the brain can change, no matter how old the person is. This offers great hope for people with dementia and those involved in their support. Psychosocial interventions are wonderful tools to enable people with dementia to stimulate their brain, and when they do so, they delay the progression of dementia. I will discuss some of the psychosocial interventions people with dementia can draw great benefit from in a later chapter.

Chapter Seven

Mental Capacity

"Power lies in the ability to choose"

What is mental capacity?

Mental capacity is the ability to make your own decisions. Let me illustrate. Let's say you want to buy a new car. You can either go to different car dealerships or look on websites on the internet where cars are being sold. You will then consider the model of the car, whether it is a small, medium or large vehicle such as a 4x4, the mileage of the car, whether it is a brand spanking new car or a second-hand one, the price, you may also consider the engine size, whether it runs on petrol, diesel, dual fuel or is electric, and you may also look at the colour of the different cars on offer. People who are into fast cars may also find out how quickly the car accelerates and whether it has fuel injection. Having sourced this information, you may also speak to someone like a mechanic who knows a lot about cars, and in particular about how easy it will be to source parts for the car, should anything breakdown (as they do from time to time), as you may not want to pay the high prices that are associated with buying cars that have been imported from another country. Armed with all the information, you may take time out to ponder what will be the best buy for you. You may do this while sipping a hot or cold drink, or some people may want to sleep on it, whilst others may need much more time to make their final decision. After all, we do not decide about buying a car rashly, as we buy a car to serve us for a considerable amount of time...no one wants to fork out on a new car every six months!

I may have laboured the point I am trying to make above, but I want to emphasise how much is involved in making important decisions. So, let us now look at what this has to do with mental capacity. For you to finally come to a decision about the car you will buy, there was a requirement for you to: receive (gather information), hold on to the information (remember), weigh up the information (compare, contrast, evaluate) and then, based on the information, come to a decision, and communicate that decision to others.

When you can do so, we say you have mental capacity. So, mental capacity is decision and time specific. With the help of our amazing brains, which are not damaged by brain injury, severe learning disabilities or a condition such as dementia, we can make our own decisions. I have to add here that this will not hold true for someone who is under the influence of drugs or alcohol, as their decision-making ability may be impaired.

Lack of mental capacity

A person may not have mental capacity because there is a problem with the way their brain functions. This is true for some people who have dementia. However, I want to hasten to add that, as mentioned previously in the chapter, mental capacity is decision and time-specific. So, someone with dementia may not be able to tell you what s/he would like to eat right now but may express their food preference five minutes later. Also, as dementia progresses, we need to enable the person with dementia to maintain their decision-making power, by presenting them with options. For example, if I asked a lady with dementia, "Which dress would you like to wear today?" she may respond: "Yes, it is a lovely warm day today!" Now whilst she may not have answered my question, her statement may indicate that she is aware of the weather and a cool dress may be her preference and not a warm woollen dress. The best thing I can do in this instance would be to hold three dresses in front of her and ask her which one she would like to wear. In this way I am empowering her to exercise the mental capacity she still has and to make decisions using this ability. Having said that, this may become increasingly difficult as dementia progresses to the more advanced stage.

When it comes to making bigger life decisions, such as whether or not to sell his or her home it may prove very difficult for someone with dementia. This is where the support of someone who has the person's best interests at heart is key. This person will then act from a position of Power of Attorney. This can be a very complicated process, especially when the relationship between family members is strained or family members are estranged and will require intervention from an unbiased, neutral person.

It is very important to note that we cannot just make assumptions that someone lacks mental capacity because of how the person looks, their age, or diagnosis. Mental capacity is something that needs to be assessed by a professional who has the tools and means to do so. We should never allow a diagnosis of dementia to determine how we approach someone with dementia. In the next chapter we will address the latter.

Chapter Eight

How to Approach Someone with Dementia

'Who am I, where am I, why am I here?'

As said in a previous chapter, dementia affects a person's daily functioning, behaviour, and memory. This can put the person with dementia in a very vulnerable position. To demonstrate, I will make use of a scenario and I want to hasten to add that the experience depicted in the scenario is not applicable to all people with dementia. We should not stereotype people with dementia.

I want you to imagine that you've just walked into a room with lots of people and you don't understand a word anyone is saying. Then you realise that you can't remember where you are or how you got there. As if this is not frightening enough, you also realise that you can't remember what your own name is. A lady in one of the care homes where we placed staff had a habit of asking: "Who am I, where am I, why am I here?" I address this in Chapter 10.

Now my question is: what will you do next? Let's say a well-meaning person, who noticed your confusion, walks up to you, and asks if you are ok and places her hand on your shoulder. You have never appreciated strangers making physical contact with you, so you push her hand off and tell her to leave you alone. She responds that she just wants to help you at which point you shout at her to go away! This draws everyone else's attention and they all look at you, frowning. How will this make you feel?

Let's say you feel that you want to get away from everyone, so start walking towards what you think is an exit and walk right into a patio door that is locked and fall to the floor. Another well-meaning person rushes over to assist you and at this point, out of sheer frustration and humiliation, you lash out and strike the person right across the face!

What should happen next? Should the police be called, and you be charged with assault? Should everyone laugh at you, or start whispering to one another about your strange behaviour? Should everyone start talking about you and not to you or just ignore you? Should they comment on how aggressive you are? What response would you want from people?

The scenario I have portrayed above could be the reality of someone with dementia. Knowing how this would affect you, I want you to consider how you respond to a person with dementia. The first and most important thing is to always maintain a person's dignity and to approach the person respecting their personal space. Just like we want people to treat us with dignity and respect, people with dementia, no matter how advanced the dementia is, deserve to be treated with the same level of dignity and respect.

The key, therefore, in approaching or interacting with someone with dementia is to do so in a sensitive way, being aware that the person may be confused, not rushing to tell the person what to do, and to speak to them in a calm, gentle and friendly tone. This may mean giving the person time to think about what they want to say, listening attentively. In Chapter 9 we will look further into communicating effectively with the person.

Chapter Nine

Effective Communication

"Non-verbal communication is still communication"

I have been working with people with dementia for almost two decades. When it comes to communication, I can probably fill this whole book with things the people whom I have worked with have shared with me. Some family members would have been embarrassed and even shocked to hear what their mum or dad have shared with me, despite a diagnosis of dementia. A very common thread has been how they are treated by their family members. Here are some examples of what had been shared with me: "She thinks I am an idiot, she speaks to me as if I am a child!"; "They think I don't understand what they are up to, plotting to put me in a care home and they've decided that I am happy with that.", "I just let her get on with it, not a word, just come here, make something for me to eat and then leave, never 'How are you feeling today mum?' "; "I've only been to their house once. I think I was too much of an inconvenience, didn't know what to do with me, just sat me in front of the telly, nothing to say."; "To some of the staff I am just a sack of potatoes."; "Sometimes I want to shout: 'You are the one who don't know what you're doing; if you did you would have treated me like a person, not something to brush off.' "

One lady, in her 80s with advanced dementia, told me in the most intricate detail how she moved from an Eastern European country to England. Her story was filled with excitement, anticipation, regret, hopelessness, shame. More poignantly, her story was filled with memories of past experiences and the most vivid, of young men who were gunned down during the war. As she described them: "They were beautiful young men."

The latter just brought another memory to my mind. I was working alongside a young man (a very snazzy dresser) in a specialist unit for people with dementia, and we were both with a lady who was bedbound, had advanced dementia and was at end of life. As I was attending to her, standing on the one side of the bed, her gaze was fixed on the young professional who was standing on the other side, with what I thought looked like great concern on her face. This lady spent most of her days sleeping, but this day she was very alert, focused and clearly had something on her mind as she stared at my colleague. On two occasions I asked her if everything was ok. I suspected that she was greatly concerned about the presence of the male person in her room. On both occasions, she turned to me and nodded but fixed her gaze straight back on the person standing on the other side of the bed. I asked her a third time if she was ok and to my surprise and sheer delight her response came; "Ain't he a fine one!!!" Now as delighted as I was that there was no issue, you can just imagine how much greater this young man's delight was to get such a compliment from someone who has been on this earth for over nine decades!

We are not able to read one another's thoughts and the worst thing we can do is to assume what someone else is thinking, or not thinking. It is therefore an absolute violation of someone with dementia's rights and dignity to think on their behalf. When given the opportunity and time to express their thoughts, people with dementia, like all of us who are able to, will share their thoughts with us. And yes, sometimes the words may not come out right, or the person may say something that makes absolutely no sense to us, but we should not use this to disempower someone from expressing themselves. There are key things to remember when communicating with someone with dementia:

- Make eye contact with the person. If the person is sitting down, pull a chair closer and sit opposite him / her or if easier, kneel down or go down on your haunches in front of him / her. However, make sure that you find out what they would prefer first.
- Show you are interested in what they have to say. This goes a very long way, especially when you ask questions about a topic the person is interested in.
- Be patient. Words may sometimes not come easily, but they will.
- When the person uses incorrect words, do not cut in and break the flow of their thought patterns. You can always remind someone that it is a watch she has on her wrist and not a doll. The connection between a watch and a doll may be the word "face", which both have. You can respond afterward with something like "What is the time on your watch please?"

- Use short uncomplicated sentences. The more advanced the dementia, the simpler sentences are, the more it will help with the flow of the conversation.
- Try to encourage conversations about what falls within the person's realm of experience and interest which will stimulate memories. This helps to get the brain cells activated, which will in turn help facilitate further conversation, and exploring new things. It is an absolute farce that people who have dementia are unable to learn new things. While they have brain cells that can be "fired up" there is an opportunity to learn. I have seen this happen over and over again. Even old skills have been brought back to life such as knitting and forming words with Scrabble blocks.

Repeating sentences

Sometimes someone with dementia may say the same thing over and over again. Instead of becoming frustrated with the person, it will be worth finding out what s/he is actually trying to tell you. As an example: someone, aged 90 may repeatedly ask to go to her mum. There is no benefit in reminding her how old she is and then asking her if she is so old, how can her mum still be alive. This can be very traumatic for the person. So, it is wise to observe when she starts asking for her mum, is it a certain time of the day, is it when something happens, or when she is simply left to sit on her own? She could be, though she does not have the words to say it, trying to tell you that she is not feeling very secure. A mum, who has been nurturing and whom she could always go to when she felt insecure in the past, therefore represents that security she is seeking, hence asking for her mum.

Behaviour is a form of communication

The term 'challenging behaviour' has become part and parcel of caring for someone with dementia, and wrongly so! When someone with dementia behaves in a way that others do not understand then the person's behaviour is described as challenging. I will provide examples. When a person with dementia lashes out and hits someone (remember the scenario I painted in Chapter 9), the person is said to be aggressive. Now we need to understand what it means when we say that someone is aggressive. Merriam-Webster dictionary states that "aggressive implies a disposition to dominate often in disregard of others' rights or in determined and energetic pursuit of one's ends." This cannot be further from the truth when referring to individuals with dementia. This is why, in practice, we refer to the person being agitated or frustrated (just like all of us get!). However, the person may not have command of the words needed to express his or her feelings, so, the s/he does something to communicate her / his frustration, by lashing out physically (because s/he still has use of her / his hand and arm).

Similarly, when someone with dementia walks back and forth in care facilities, or for some, even at home, they are labelled as "wandering". This happens frequently when someone with dementia is left sitting on their own for long periods of time, without any physical stimulation or social engagement. We all (well most of us, apart from those who enjoy just lazing around, day in, day out) feel the need to do something most days, to have a sense of purpose or occupation. This is no different for someone with dementia; this need does not vanish into thin air just because someone has dementia. People still need to feel that they have a reason to get up in the morning and have a contribution to make; this could be from dusting furniture to making furniture or anything else that has nothing to do with furniture. I trust you get my point.

Chapter Ten

Person-centred Support

"The person is at the centre of what we do"

It is very important to recognise that in all care settings we are caring for people, not a disease like Alzheimer's, cancer, or tuberculosis. The person comes first, then the condition. It is critical to remember this when caring for someone with dementia. Too often, the main focus can be on the dementia and then the personhood of the individual is lost. It is therefore important that we place the person at the centre of all we do.

In practice, this starts with history taking. We consider the biology of the person; their health, their routines including exercise and eating habits, any health conditions that they have / had, any dependencies they may have / had such as an alcohol dependency, prescription medication, what abilities they have, including those developed through previous careers and development and so on. We then consider the emotional wellbeing of the person, whether they had any trauma in their lives or any mental health challenges. Next, we explore things such as the person's support networks, including family and friends, what social engagement the person enjoys, what the person's hobbies are / were previously. Once we have built this picture of the 'whole person', we are able to put a plan of care in place that will best meet the person's needs, identifying the key role players who will have to be involved to facilitate this, from the GP to care worker and everyone in between, including and not limited to speech and language therapists, social workers, occupational therapist, chiropodist and the list goes on and on. The care plan is amended on an ongoing basis, as the person's needs change. This is the only way to ensure person-centred support.

In delivering person-centred support, there are key principles that we need to apply. These are:

- Maintaining the person's **dignity**
- Treating the person with **respect**

- Upholding the **rights** of the person
- Offering **choice**
- Promoting the person's **individuality**
- Enabling the person to maintain their **independence**
- Maintaining **privacy**
- Fostering **partnership** working
- Protecting **confidentiality**

When we apply these principles in caring for someone with dementia, we are more likely to be effective in what we do and in doing so will enhance the person's well-being and overall quality of life.

Chapter Eleven

Psychosocial Interventions

"Remaining engaged is key"

Psychosocial interventions involve a variety of ways to support people to overcome life-changing challenges and to maintain good mental health, without the use of medication. These interventions or therapies, as they are sometimes called, are available to people with dementia and their family members. Whilst, for the person who has dementia, there is a great focus on stimulating their brain (cognitive function), the therapies also provide great opportunities for social engagement, physical stimulation, and nurturing existing skills and talents, while learning new ones. I want to repeat and emphasise here that people with dementia are able to learn new things, despite having the condition. Therapies also give people with dementia and their family members opportunities to enjoy activities together.

There are several psychosocial interventions offered to people with dementia and their families. However, access will depend on where you live and the availability of trained facilitators. The possibility of joining sessions remotely, via a video-link, increases the scope of finding sessions to join. This option will involve having a reliable internet connection.

Some of the therapies that have evidence of being very beneficial are:

Animal-assisted therapy

Animal-assisted therapy involves having access to animals for the purpose of improving wellbeing and quality of life. A good example of this is petting farms, both those that people can visit or mobile petting farms that travel to where people live. This form of therapy gives people with dementia (and their family carers) a great opportunity to get in close contact with animals by holding and stroking them, which offers great sensory stimulation, so it is very therapeutic in that it creates a "feel-good" experience. However, it is important to note that animal-assisted therapy is different from caring for a pet at home, as it involves specific goals and outcomes. Contact with animals takes place under the supervision of a trained handler, who facilitates the interaction with the animal. In some instances, animal-assisted therapy involves having an animal stay over at an individual's home. This may occur where there is a need for companionship or to improve someone's mood, wellbeing or to help someone connect with the outside world.

I have seen how the experiences gained during these sessions in care facilities created great topics for discussions afterwards. Let's face it, it's not an everyday experience to get close and handle a beautiful creature such as a snowy owl or a fluffy Angora rabbit. I've even witnessed the faint-hearted becoming bold enough to handle a snake.

Creative arts therapies

Creative arts therapies are forms of treatment for people with dementia that use paints, stories, poetry, crafts, music, and several other media. It has a therapeutic focus and differ from general art activities. It offers several benefits to individuals who experience emotional difficulties and promotes enhanced quality of life. Sessions can be delivered on an individual basis or in a group. It is a great way to get individuals to express their own thoughts, ideas, opinions, and emotions which are difficult to express in words.

Cognitive Stimulation Therapy and Maintenance Cognitive Stimulation Therapy

Cognitive stimulation therapy (CST) is a group therapy that is delivered by a trained CST practitioner. It is used to slow down cognitive decline and to help strengthen a person's communications skills, thinking and memory. It is suitable for people with a diagnosis of mild to moderate dementia. CST groups run for a limited number of sessions, ideally twice per week and if not possible, once a week. It involves a range of group activities and exercises designed to help maintain memory and mental functioning such as problem solving, as well as improve language ability. Social functioning is an important aspect of CST, and participants are expected to engage and work with other group members. A wide range of activities such as discussions of past events, current news, other topics of interest, word games, puzzles, activities involving music, such as singing along or clapping using rhythmic patterns, as well as practical activities such as flower arranging, gardening, or painting with numbers all form part of CST.

There is a lot of research that provides evidence that CST improves wellbeing and quality of life. This is not surprising, as participants benefit from improvements in cognitive function and communication with others, which boost their self-esteem and self-confidence.

A number of years ago I lead a CST pilot programme for a branch of the UK's largest charity that support older people and witnessed first-hand how these sessions boosted the self-confidence of those who attended. More so, the friendships and bonds that developed stretched beyond the sessions.

Maintenance cognitive stimulation therapy (MCST) groups continue indefinitely and aim to maintain the benefits that CST groups provide.

Cognitive rehabilitation

Cognitive rehabilitation is an approach to managing the impact that dementia-related challenges, such as difficulties with memory and thinking, can have on a person's daily life. It can involve learning strategies for managing memory problems, or better ways of tackling everyday tasks. Sometimes people choose to learn something new, such as how to use a mobile phone or iPad, to help in everyday situations, or to resume activities they used to enjoy. Cognitive rehabilitation is not about correcting or reducing dementia-related difficulties with thinking and memory; rather it is about learning ways of compensating for these difficulties or managing them better. It is suitable for people who have early-stage dementia and programmes often involve family members and carers. It involves a process whereby the person with dementia identifies aspects of their lives they would like to improve upon or manage better. This will involve a discussion with a trained professional, during which an agreement is reached about the goals they will work towards together. The professional will then provide support to find ways of achieving the goals.

Cognitive training

As mentioned previously, the brain is neuroplastic, meaning it can be changed. Cognitive training assumes that the brain is like a muscle and can benefit from regular exercise to stay healthy ('brain training'). It also assumes that if you have dementia, you can maintain your current level of functioning or slow down decline through training your brain. The 'brain training' involves taking part in games such as those played on electronic devices, completing crossword puzzles or Sudoku, to name a few. The approach involves engaging in these activities daily for a set period of time, with the aim of enhancing specific functions of the brain, such as thinking skills, reasoning, word recall and image recognition. Cognitive training activities need to be continued to maintain the benefits. Cognitive training is for anyone, including people with dementia, who wants to keep their brain active and enjoys brain training games and puzzles.

Dementia café or memory café

Dementia cafés or memory cafés are group meetings that run on an informal basis, open to people with dementia and those involved in their support. It operates on a drop-in basis. These gatherings are places where people with dementia, family members, carers and professionals can meet together to share information and experiences and speak openly about dementia. Anyone else, who has an interest in dementia or wants to learn more about dementia, is also welcome to drop in. The purpose of these groups is to provide a platform where people can talk openly and informally about dementia, sharing their knowledge, experience and expertise while having a hot drink together. It aims to reduce the social isolation of people who are impacted by dementia, such as those with dementia and their family members or carers.

Life story work

Life story work involves looking back on the past and recording important personal events, as well as looking forward to things individuals hope for in the future. It usually involves one-to-one work with a spouse, family members or someone who can guide the couple through the process. It can also be done with a professional. Life story work is the process of remembering and recording past events and memories so that a biography is created. It is used to help a person with dementia to remember past events and to communicate and share these memories and future hopes with other people. A life storybook often contains photographs or pictures which can help to illustrate the person's memories and important moments. If preferred, the end product of life story work can also be in the form of a website, video presentation, a brief time-line, tapestry, soundtrack, or scrapbook. It is a lovely way to create an autobiographical story of an individual's life.

I have seen family members benefiting greatly from what becomes an invaluable family treasure, knowing that their loved one left them something to remember them by; something authentic, unique and tailor-made, showcasing the tenacity of the human spirit, albeit a diagnosis of dementia.

Music therapy

Music therapy describes interventions that use music and music-based therapeutic activities to improve the wellbeing of people with dementia. It involves a qualified music therapist using a range of specialist approaches to help people with dementia to explore their emotions. The therapy can also form part of reminiscence, to help bring old memories to the surface. The therapy can be offered to an individual or in a group. Group sessions are great, as it offers opportunities for social engagement and sharing music interests with others. It involves singing together and using musical instruments to create music together. Music therapy is very effective in enhancing individuals' wellbeing and quality of life, as it promotes mental wellbeing.

I have been astounded by the changes in participants' emotional wellbeing when engaging in this intervention. Individuals who hardly said a word for weeks were suddenly bellowing songs they recognised from the top of their lungs or jumping to their feet to dance...two ladies, in particular, swaying their hips to "When the saints go marching in!" It is the most joyous and precious thing to observe and a great source of encouragement of what can be done to improve individuals' overall quality of life. An added benefit is the endorphins (happy hormones) that are released when individuals have so much fun.

Reminiscence

Reminiscence is an activity that involves people with dementia remembering and retelling memories and events from their personal experiences. The sessions often involve the use of materials from a particular time. It is more general than, and different from, life story work. This therapy is suited for anyone with a diagnosis of dementia and takes place in a group setting in which people share memories and listen to one another. Reminiscence offers people with dementia opportunities to revisit familiar times and share common experiences with others in the group. Photos, music, and objects from a particular point in time are used to jog individuals' memory. The therapy focuses on accessing an individual with dementia's preserved memory, thereby stimulating cognitive function. Discussions often centre around memories of childhood, school days, specific locations such as neighbourhoods, towns, and cities, family favourites, and specific events that individuals can identify with, such as getting their first telephone, car, or television, following themes. The therapy sessions are a great opportunity for people with dementia to engage socially, thereby enhancing their wellbeing and quality of life.

Chapter Twelve

Support and Advice

"A problem shared is a problem halved"

Obtaining guidance from a dementia advisor is key to finding the right support, whether you or someone close to you show signs of having dementia, have a diagnosis of dementia or support someone living with dementia. You can get support from different people or organisations as described below.

Dementia Adviser

A dementia adviser is someone who can provide ongoing support to enable someone to live well with dementia. A dementia adviser can support a person with dementia, their family members and close friends who are involved in their support and care. A key role of the dementia adviser is to provide information the person needs, at a time when it is needed and to help someone access what they need. For example, if an agreement has been reached with the person who has dementia that it is necessary for a caregiver to support them with their daily medication, then a dementia adviser can assist to search for organisations who place caregivers, find out if the caregivers have the qualities and skills needed, when they are available to start and sit in during an interview meeting to ensure the right person is placed.

It is important to note that it is not the role of the dementia adviser to make decision about someone's life, but rather to empower all involved with the tools they need to maintain overall wellbeing and quality of life. It is important, as far as possible to contact a dementia adviser well in advance, before reaching a critical point, to ensure that assistance can be sourced in a timely manner. Appointments can take place face-to-face, via a phone call or video chat.

Dementia advisers help individuals to work their way through the journey of dementia and can be great sources who offer encouragement, knowledge about dementia and care support, helping to reduce uncertainty, anxiety, and burnout in the case of caregivers.

Post-diagnostic courses

Post-diagnostic courses which focus on the topic of dementia are a great way for people with dementia and those involved in their care to be empowered with knowledge and skills about dementia. As mentioned in Chapter 2, not all people will have the same experience of dementia, as there are so many types of dementia, each presenting its own symptoms. There are just so many things to consider. However, there will be similarities and it is these commonalities which, when understood, can be addressed in a group setting such as a training course. To give an example: because of memory loss, some people with dementia may forget how to eat, so may sit looking at the food. A training session can cover practical ways of empowering the person to eat. These sessions are a great place to ask questions, receive knowledge and practical guidance. Learning from people who have dementia during sessions is an invaluable resource in getting insight into the lived experience of dementia.

Post-diagnostic groups

Post-diagnostic groups offer a great source of support to people who receive a diagnosis of dementia, as well as for their family members and close friends who are involved in their support. These groups run regular sessions and invite speakers who will deliver talks around the topic of dementia. Sometimes these groups are referred to as post-diagnostic support or memory groups.

These groups offer the opportunity to meet with people who may face similar challenges in dealing with dementia. It is also a great place to find out how they are managing some of the challenges, what has worked well, and what remains challenging, so that a group effort can be made to address the issue.

Having moral support from others can truly have an immense impact on someone's experience, and reduces feelings of being alone, isolated, and uninformed, therefore powerless, but rather feeling included, supported and empowered to live well with dementia (which is very possible), or to support someone with dementia in the most caring, compassionate, competent and confident way.

Post-Diagnostic Counselling

Post-diagnostic counselling is a supportive process to help people with dementia and those closest to them to come to terms with the diagnosis. These sessions help individuals to talk through feelings, including fears and uncertainties about the future. Moreover, it is to help people consider the various options available to them and how to access these in a manageable, structured, and organised way, dealing with things methodically, as to prevent them from becoming overwhelmed or stressed. As much as the sessions are designed to help someone come to terms with a diagnosis of dementia, other topics such as how and when to share this information with others and making decisions about the future such as advanced care planning, in other words, putting things in place for when the condition progresses.

The most effective sessions are delivered by a trained counsellor who has extensive experience working with people with dementia and those involved in their support. This service is usually available at a memory clinic, but an independent specialist dementia consultant, who is highly qualified in the area of dementia, can also assist in this regard.

Family therapy

Family therapy is a form of psychotherapy that involves helping people who are in a close relationship with each other to understand each other and communicate their feelings and emotions to each other. It is for people with dementia and their families. Receiving a diagnosis of dementia can have a profound impact on the person receiving the diagnosis and those close to them. It can place great strain on the relationship, especially when they don't have the knowledge and understanding of how to live well with dementia. Family therapy aims to improve understanding between people in close relationships and to help people to communicate their feelings to one another. Family therapy sessions are designed to provide individuals with a safe place to express themselves. The therapy involves people talking openly about the current issues and feelings and listening to one another. The therapist can help individuals to learn better ways of relating to one another and how they may be able to help one another during times of difficulty. Family therapy aims to improve the wellbeing of individuals who have dementia and the wellbeing of those close to them.

Care / Social Farming

Care farming (or social farming as it is sometimes known) can be understood as the 'therapeutic use of farming practices'. Care farms deliver services for individuals from one or a range of vulnerable groups of people, including people with dementia. Services are run from farms and provide programmes of farming-related activities. The support provided is supervised, structured and bespoke, and delivered on a regular basis for service users.

Care farms can be found in many countries around the world, but particularly in Holland where they are part of mainstream health and social care services for people with dementia and have been around for decades. In the UK (2024) there are approximately 300 care farms with roughly 75 delivering regular services to those living with dementia.

People with dementia attend care farms for many reasons. For example, for social contact, an interest in animals, horticulture, a work type experience or because they want to help others. The farm setting can be helpful in supporting people with dementia to have meaningful experiences and to maintain the status in society of someone who is useful.

One of my close friends and a respected colleague, Justin Mazzotta, the director of Beetle Bank Social Farm in York, England, is committed to growing this effective type of intervention in the UK. To find out more about the work Justin and his team do, visit their website: https://www.beetlebanksocialfarm.org

Justin is also a trusted cognitive rehabilitation therapist.

enABLE Foundation

*en*ABLE Foundation is a non-profit organisation committed to helping reduce the impact of dementia.

The organisation supports individuals with dementia and those involved in their care and support, such as family members and health and social care professionals, to enhance the quality of life of people with dementia holistically. This is achieved through sharing information, i.e., advocacy and education, as well as through offering practical support. To this end, enABLE Foundation helps to create a greater understanding of dementia, including how dementia can be prevented. The organisation signposts those who may have concerns relating to signs and symptoms of dementia, those who have dementia, as well as those who are involved in the care and support of people with dementia, to services and resources to enable individuals to live well with dementia. Moreover, it empowers others with knowledge and skills about dementia, to help reduce the stigma associated with dementia. enABLE Foundation is actively involved in research in the area of dementia and constantly seeks to influence dementia strategies and policies to promote better outcomes for people with dementia and those involved in their care and support.

The organisation applies research-based practice, centred on extensive research carried out by people who have had a significant impact on the way people with dementia are viewed, treated, and supported.

enABLE Foundation offers consultancy, training, and support in ways that are most effective in addressing the issue of dementia.

More information about the organisation can be found on its website: www.enablefoundation.org

I sincerely trust that you now not only have a much clearer understanding of dementia but also recognise how people who are impacted by dementia can be supported effectively, in a person-centred way, to enhance their wellbeing and quality of life. I want to challenge you to use the knowledge you've acquired through reading this book, to act as an ambassador and agent of change to promote dementia-friendly communities. You can do this by empowering others and helping to reduce the stigma associated with dementia by standing up against the stereotypes others have about it.

Just for your benefit, please consider completing the quiz again if you attempted it before you started reading. Or, if you have not completed it previously.

ALL THE BEST!!

QUIZ

Chapter One

1. Dementia is a disease.

   TRUE / FALSE

2. Alzheimer's disease is very different from dementia.

   TRUE / FALSE

3. There are over 200 different types of dementia.

   TRUE / FALSE

4. There is currently no cure for dementia.

   TRUE / FALSE

5. Not much can be done for people who have dementia.

   TRUE / FALSE

6. The first sign of dementia, in anyone who develops it, is forgetting things.

TRUE / FALSE

7. People with dementia are not able to make their own decisions at all.

TRUE / FALSE

8. Someone develops dementia because they have been bewitched.

TRUE / FALSE

9. Only people over the age of 65 develop dementia.

TRUE / FALSE

10. People with dementia can still live a very productive life but may need support with some things.

TRUE / FALSE

11. Dementia affects both men and women.

TRUE / FALSE

12. It is impossible for a 40-year-old person to develop dementia.

TRUE / FALSE

Chapter Two

1. Alzheimer's disease affects 60-70% of people who have dementia.

   TRUE / FALSE

2. Alzheimer's disease causes 'plaques' and 'tangles' in the brain cells.

   TRUE / FALSE

3. When someone has dementia their brain cells shrink, and eventually die.

   TRUE / FALSE

4. Dementia is progressive, meaning more and more brain cells become affected as time goes on.

   TRUE / FALSE

5. Someone who had a stroke is not a risk of developing dementia.

   TRUE / FALSE

6. Lewy Body dementia is often mistaken for Alzheimer's disease.

   TRUE / FALSE

7. Frontotemporal dementia only affects one part of the brain.

   TRUE / FALSE

8. When someone has more than one type of dementia, we say the person has mixed dementia.

   TRUE / FALSE

9. Drinking heavily over long periods does not put someone at risk of developing dementia.

   TRUE / FALSE

10. A person who has HIV or AIDS is at risk of developing dementia.

    TRUE / FALSE

Chapter Three

1. All people with dementia have the same symptoms.

   TRUE / FALSE

2. Some people with dementia may take longer to complete their usual daily tasks.

   TRUE / FALSE

3. Someone with dementia may find planning or solving problems difficult.

   TRUE / FALSE

4. If someone who has dementia does not pay their bills, it means that they want to save their money.

   TRUE / FALSE

5. A person with dementia may repeat themselves because they want to irritate others, especially their family members.

TRUE / FALSE

6. If a person with dementia calls someone else by the wrong name, you can point out that they may have dementia.

   TRUE / FALSE

7. When someone with Lewy body dementia starts seeing animals and people who are not there, it is a sign that they are bewitched.

   TRUE / FALSE

8. Depression and anxiety are commonly seen in people who have Lewy body dementia, but they can receive treatment.

   TRUE / FALSE

9. When someone is confused and has problems with her/his balance, it is a sure sign that s/he has dementia.

   TRUE / FALSE

10. Someone with dementia will make inappropriate jokes or show inappropriate sexual behaviour because they just want to upset others.

    TRUE / FALSE

11. Individuals with dementia may not realise that they are experiencing changes in their personality or behaviour, but the changes can become very upsetting to family members.

TRUE / FALSE

12. It is very important to seek professional advice as soon as you or someone close to you start showing signs of dementia that are persistent and increase in frequency.

TRUE / FALSE

Chapter Four

1. It is easy to decide if someone has dementia, you can just check if they are forgetting things.

   TRUE / FALSE

2. It is better to wait at least one year before getting professional help when someone shows signs of dementia.

   TRUE / FALSE

3. People with dementia do not usually experience stigma, as others are very supportive.

   TRUE / FALSE

4. If you notice someone has symptoms of dementia, it is best to tell them that they have dementia straight away and there is no need to seek advice from a professional first, as it is easy to spot dementia.

   TRUE / FALSE

5. Someone who shows signs of dementia will not be able to make their own decisions, so it is best to start making their decisions for them as soon as possible.

   TRUE / FALSE

6. It is possible that someone has a urine infection when the person shows signs of being confused.

   TRUE / FALSE

7. A neurologist can tell us if we have dementia.

   TRUE / FALSE

8. It is good for someone who has difficulty remembering things to visit a memory clinic.

   TRUE / FALSE

9. There is no need to get different health professionals involved when someone shows signs of having dementia. A doctor will be able to meet all the person's health needs.

   TRUE / FALSE

10. An occupational therapist can help someone to find work.

    TRUE / FALSE

11. There is no need to know someone's medical history before diagnosing the person with dementia.

TRUE / FALSE

12. Someone with dementia may need the help of a care worker as the dementia progresses.

TRUE / FALSE

Chapter Five

1. No medication is specifically available for dementia, so it is best to give people with dementia anti-depressants or sleeping tablets to help them manage their symptoms.

   TRUE / FALSE

2. We don't need to discuss medication options with people with dementia and their family members as they are not medically trained.

   TRUE / FALSE

3. There is currently no medication to cure dementia. However, the right medication can play an important role in helping to manage the symptoms of dementia.

   TRUE / FALSE

4. Giving someone with dementia sleeping tablets to control their behaviour is a form of abuse.

   TRUE / FALSE

5. It is best to hide medication in food when giving it to someone with dementia.

TRUE / FALSE

6. Whenever medication is prescribed to someone with dementia, consideration should be given to other medicines the person takes.

TRUE / FALSE

7. It is important that those who are involved in making decisions on behalf of someone who lacks capacity have the person's best interest at heart.

TRUE / FALSE

8. Although there is no medication to cure dementia, there is medication to slow down its progress.

TRUE / FALSE

9. Dementia medication helps improve the person's functioning and well-being.

TRUE / FALSE

10. Medication given to someone with dementia should improve the person's quality of life.

TRUE / FALSE

Chapter Six

1. Our brains cannot be changed after we reach the age of 60.

   TRUE / FALSE

2. The brain is only responsible for helping us think.

   TRUE / FALSE

3. Dementia is caused by damage to someone's brain.

   TRUE / FALSE

4. The human brain is divided into a forebrain, midbrain and hindbrain.

   TRUE / FALSE

5. If someone's frontal lobe of their brain is damaged it affects their behaviour, planning and decision-making

   TRUE / FALSE

6. Damage to the temporal lobe of someone's brain will cause them to forget things.

   TRUE / FALSE

7. The part of the brain that controls vision is at the back of the head.

   TRUE / FALSE

8. If someone with dementia calls her/his daughter by their mum's name, then it is because the s/he is missing her/his mum.

   TRUE / FALSE

9. Left-handed people only use the left side of their brains.

   TRUE / FALSE

10. The left and right sides of the brain operate independently and don't need to work together.

    TRUE / FALSE

Chapter Seven

1. To have mental capacity means we can make our own decisions.

   TRUE / FALSE

2. Mental capacity is decision and time-specific.

   TRUE / FALSE

3. All people with dementia do not have mental capacity.

   TRUE / FALSE

4. Damage to someone's brain may affect their ability to make their own decisions.

   TRUE / FALSE

5. Someone who has Power of Attorney can support a person with dementia when making a big decision such as selling a property.

   TRUE / FALSE

6. If someone has dementia, s/he will not be able to tell you what s/he would like for supper, so there is no point asking her/him.

   TRUE / FALSE

7. If someone with dementia gives an answer that appears unrelated to the question, it means that the person does not have any idea what you are talking about.

   TRUE / FALSE

8. Mental capacity may decrease in someone who has Alzheimer's disease.

   TRUE / FALSE

9. We cannot make assumptions about someone's mental capacity based on the person's age or appearance.

   TRUE / FALSE

10. Mental capacity needs to be assessed by a professional who is qualified to do so.

    TRUE / FALSE

Chapter Eight

1. Individuals who have dementia can become very vulnerable to being mistreated.

   TRUE / FALSE

2. We need to engage with someone who has dementia in a sensitive way; respecting the person's personal space and promoting their dignity.

   TRUE / FALSE

3. When someone who has dementia does something inappropriate it is ok to laugh at him/her.

   TRUE / FALSE

4. It is ok to leave someone with dementia out of the conversation, even if s/he is sitting with us, as the person does not understand what we are talking about.

TRUE / FALSE

5. Someone may behave in a way that is seen as inappropriate when s/he feels insecure.

   TRUE / FALSE

6. People who have dementia lose their sense of direction all the time.

   TRUE / FALSE

7. We need to treat someone who has dementia like a child because people with dementia become like children.

   TRUE / FALSE

8. We should never assume that a person with dementia doesn't understand what is going on around them.

   TRUE / FALSE

9. We must never assume that we know better than someone who has dementia.

   TRUE / FALSE

10. Respecting someone who has dementia is as important as respecting those who don't.

    TRUE / FALSE

Chapter Nine

1. We should give people who have dementia time to express their thoughts.

   TRUE / FALSE

2. It is not necessary to make eye contact with someone who has dementia as the person may not recognise who you are.

   TRUE / FALSE

3. We can talk to others about someone who has dementia in their presence as the person won't understand what we are saying.

   TRUE / FALSE

4. We need to wait patiently for someone with dementia to express themselves, even when their dementia is at an advanced stage.

   TRUE / FALSE

5. It is best to correct someone with dementia immediately when they use the wrong word.

TRUE / FALSE

6. It is best to use easy, short sentences when talking with someone who has dementia.

TRUE / FALSE

7. We must always show an interest in what someone with dementia tells us even if we think what they talk about is nonsense.

TRUE / FALSE

8. When someone who has dementia says something over and over again it is because they only remember a few words.

TRUE / FALSE

9. When a 90-year-old lady asks for her mum, it is best to remind her that her mum passed away a long time ago.

TRUE / FALSE

10. Behaviour is a form of communication.

TRUE / FALSE

Chapter Ten

1. A person-centred approach means we put the person at the centre of all the support we give him.

   TRUE / FALSE

2. It doesn't matter how we speak to someone with dementia because they don't understand us anyway.

   TRUE / FALSE

3. People who develop dementia should lose all their rights in society.

   TRUE / FALSE

4. It is ok to refer to people who have dementia as being like children because they are.

   TRUE / FALSE

5. We don't need to know someone's history before

we start caring for them, as we just take each day as it comes.

TRUE / FALSE

6. It is not relevant to know if someone with dementia drank a lot in the past when we care for them.

   TRUE / FALSE

7. Knowing what someone did for a career can help us to plan their care.

   TRUE / FALSE

8. It is important that someone is supported to maintain as much independence as possible when we provide care for the person.

   TRUE / FALSE

9. We can share information about the person we support with anyone who asks for it.

   TRUE / FALSE

10. We don't have to offer people with dementia choices of what to eat or wear. We can decide for them.

    TRUE / FALSE

11. Someone who can't talk has no way of telling us what they would like to wear or eat.

TRUE / FALSE

12. We can wash someone who has dementia in front of others as they don't understand that others may be watching.

TRUE / FALSE

Chapter Eleven

1. People with dementia can only improve their lives with the help of medication that makes them sleep.

   TRUE / FALSE

2. Anyone, even if not trained, can offer support sessions to someone who has dementia and their family members, as it is not difficult to do.

   TRUE / FALSE

3. We can just use what we've experienced with a few people who have dementia to know how to support others, as they all have the same challenges.

   TRUE / FALSE

4. Animal-assisted therapy means having your own pet at home to take care of.

   TRUE / FALSE

5. It is best for someone who has dementia to stay indoors so that they don't embarrass themselves and others.

   TRUE / FALSE

6. Someone with dementia cannot learn new things so there is no point in joining any new activities.

   TRUE / FALSE

7. Creative art therapy is a great way for people with dementia to express what they feel and think.

   TRUE / FALSE

8. Problem-solving activities help people with dementia to keep their minds active.

   TRUE / FALSE

9. Some people with dementia can boost their confidence by taking part in group sessions that are specifically developed to meet their needs.

   TRUE / FALSE

10. The brain is like a muscle that needs regular exercise to stay healthy.

    TRUE / FALSE

11. Dementia cafés sell food for people who have dementia.

TRUE / FALSE

12. It is not good for people with dementia to talk about the past as it could mean that they are trapped in it.

TRUE / FALSE

Chapter Twelve

1. A dementia advisor can offer support to family members of someone who has dementia.

   TRUE / FALSE

2. A dementia advisor can diagnose someone with dementia.

   TRUE / FALSE

3. Caregivers are best able to decide if someone has dementia, even if they are not medically trained, because they spend a lot of time with the person.

   TRUE / FALSE

4. It is best to wait as long as possible before contacting a dementia advisor, as they are very busy, and it is not good to take up their time when you're not sure if someone has dementia.

   TRUE / FALSE

5. People who have dementia can teach us more about the condition.

TRUE / FALSE

6. There is no need to attend training about dementia as not much is known about it.

TRUE / FALSE

7. Counselling can help the person who has a diagnosis of dementia to come to terms with it.

TRUE / FALSE

8. Memory groups are a good place for family members and close friends of someone with dementia to share their experiences, learn from others, and get moral support.

TRUE / FALSE

9. Family therapy offers great opportunities for family members to talk through their feelings and to help understand one another.

TRUE / FALSE

10. Anyone can offer advise about dementia, without being trained to do so.

TRUE / FALSE

ANSWERS

Chapter 1

1. FALSE
2. FALSE
3. TRUE
4. TRUE
5. FALSE
6. FALSE
7. FALSE
8. FALSE
9. FALSE
10. TRUE
11. TRUE
12. FALSE

Chapter 2

1. TRUE
2. TRUE
3. TRUE
4. TRUE
5. FALSE
6. TRUE
7. FALSE
8. FALSE
9. TRUE
10. FALSE

Chapter 3

1. FALSE
2. TRUE
3. TRUE
4. FALSE
5. FALSE
6. FALSE
7. FALSE
8. TRUE
9. FALSE
10. FALSE
11. TRUE
12. TRUE

Chapter 4

1. FALSE
2. FALSE
3. FALSE
4. FALSE
5. FALSE
6. TRUE
7. TRUE
8. TRUE
9. FALSE
10. FALSE
11. FALSE
12. TRUE

Chapter 5

1. FALSE
2. FALSE
3. TRUE
4. TRUE
5. FALSE
6. TRUE
7. TRUE
8. TRUE
9. TRUE
10. TRUE

Chapter 6

1. FALSE
2. FALSE
3. TRUE
4. TRUE
5. TRUE
6. TRUE
7. TRUE
8. FALSE
9. FALSE
10. FALSE

Chapter 7

1. TRUE
2. TRUE
3. FALSE
4. TRUE
5. TRUE
6. FALSE
7. FALSE
8. TRUE
9. TRUE
10. TRUE

Chapter 8

1. TRUE
2. TRUE
3. FALSE
4. FALSE
5. TRUE
6. FALSE
7. FALSE
8. TRUE
9. TRUE
10. TRUE

Chapter 9

1. TRUE
2. FALSE
3. FALSE
4. TRUE
5. FALSE
6. TRUE
7. TRUE
8. FALSE
9. FALSE
10. TRUE

Chapter 10

1. TRUE
2. FALSE
3. FALSE
4. FALSE
5. FALSE
6. FALSE
7. TRUE
8. TRUE
9. FALSE
10. FALSE
11. FALSE
12. FALSE

Chapter 11

1. FALSE
2. FALSE
3. FALSE
4. FALSE
5. FALSE
6. FALSE
7. TRUE
8. TRUE
9. TRUE
10. TRUE
11. FALSE
12. FALSE

Chapter 12

1. TRUE
2. FALSE
3. FALSE
4. FALSE
5. TRUE
6. FALSE
7. TRUE
8. TRUE
9. TRUE
10. FALSE

Record your scores here:

	First attempt	Second attempt
Chapter 1		
Chapter 2		
Chapter 3		
Chapter 4		
Chapter 5		
Chapter 6		
Chapter 7		
Chapter 8		
Chapter 9		
Chapter 10		
Chapter 11		
Chapter 12		
TOTAL	/130	/130

BIBLIOGRAPHY

Aggressive." Merriam-Webster.com Dictionary, Merriam-Webster, https://www.merriam-webster.com/dictionary/aggressive. Accessed15 February 2023.

Alzheimers Disease International (2020). Dementiastatistics. https://www.alzint.org/about/dementia-facts-figures/dementia-statistics/

Brooker, D. (2007). Person-centred dementia care. *Making services better.* Jessica Kingsley Publishers.

Burnham, M. (2009). Memory groups for people with early dementia. In E. Moniz-Cook, E. and J, Manthorpe, J. (Eds). *Early interventions in dementia. Evidence-based practice.* Jessica Kingsley Publishers.

Cheston, R. (2009). Group psychotherapy for people with early dementia. In E. Moniz-Cook, and J, Manthorpe (Eds). *Early interventions in dementia. Evidence-based practice.* Jessica Kingsley Publishers.

Clare, L. (2008). Neurological rehabilitation and people with dementia. *Neuropsychological rehabilitation: A Modular Handbook*. Psychology Press.

Cohen-Mansfield, J. (2014).Understanding behaviour. In M, Downs and B, Bowers (Eds). *Excellence in dementia care. Research into practice.* (2nd ed.) Open University Press.

Downs, M., Clare, L., & Anderson, E. (2008).Dementia as a biopsychosocial condition: Implications for practice and research In R. T. Woods & L. Clare (Eds.) *Handbook of the clinical psychology of ageing* (2nd ed.) Chichester: John Wiley & Sons Ltd.

enABLE Foundation. www.enablefoundation.org

Folkerts, A.K *et al.* (2018). 'Cognitive Stimulation for Individuals with Parkinson's Disease Dementia Living in Long-Term Care: Preliminary Data from a Randomised Crossover Pilot Study', *Parkinson's Disease (20420080),* pp. 1-9 doi: 10.1155/2018/8104673.

Harmer, B. J., & Orrell, M. (2008). What is meaningful activity for people with dementia living in care homes? A comparison of the views of older people with dementia, staff and family carers. *Aging & Mental Health*, *12*, 548 – 558. doi:10.1080/13607860802343019

Kitwood, T. (1997). *Dementia reconsidered: The person comes first.* Buckingham: Open University Press.

Lokon, E., Sauer, P.E. and Li, Y. (2019) 'Activities in dementia care: A comparative assessment of activity types', *Dementia (14713012),* 18(2), pp. 471-489. doi: 10.1177/1471301216680890.

Menne, H. L., Johnson, J. D., Whitlatch, C. J., & Schwartz, S. M. (2012). Activity preferences of persons with dementia. *Activities, Adaptation & Aging, 36,* 195–213. doi:10.1080/01924788.201 2.696234

Merriam-Webster's Collegiate Dictionary (10th ed.). (2023). Merriam-Webster Incorporated.

Moniz-Cook, E *et al.* (2009). Timely psychosocial interventions in a memory clinic. In E. Moniz-Cook, and J, Manthorpe (Eds). *Early interventions in dementia. Evidence-based practice.* Jessica Kingsley Publishers.

National Institute for Health and Clinical Excellence (2011). Donepesil, galantamine, rivistigmine and memantine for the treatment of Alzheimer's disease. NICE technology appraisal guidance 217. http//guidance.nice.org.uk/TA217

Orrell, M. *et al.* (2014) 'Maintenance cognitive stimulation therapy for dementia: single-blind, multicentre, pragmatic randomised controlled trial', *British Journal of Psychiatry*, 204(6), pp. 454-461. doi: 10.1192/bjp.bp.113.137414.

Oyebode, J and Clare, L.(2008). Supporting cognitive abilities. In M, Downs and B, Bowers (Eds). *Excellence in dementia care. Research into practice.* Open University Press.

Phinney, A. (2008). Towards understanding subjective experiences of dementia. In M, Downs and B, Bowers (Eds). *Excellence in dementia care. Research into practice.* Open University Press,pp 35-47.

Sabat, S.R.(2008).A bio-psycho-social approach to dementia.In M, Downs and B, Bowers (Eds). *Excellence in dementia care. Research into practice.* Open University Press, pp. 70-84.

Spectre A, Orrell, M and Woods, B. (2010).Cognitive Stimulation Therapy (CST): effects on different areas of cognitive function for people with dementia: International Journal of Geriatric Psychiatry, 25 (12): 1253 - 1258.

Whitlatch, C,J.(2014) Understanding and enhancing the relationship between people with dementia and their family carers. In M, Downs and B, Bowers (Eds). *Excellence in dementia care. Research into practice.* (2nd ed.) Open University Press.

Woods B, Aquirre E, Spector A.E, Orrell M (2012). Cognitive stimulation to improve cognitive functioning in people with dementia.*Cochraine Database of Systematic Reviews:* CD005562

World Health Organization (2018).Towards a dementia plan: a WHO guide. Geneva: Licence: CC BY-NC-SA 3.0 IGO.

BLURB

With over 55 million people worldwide currently living with dementia, of which 60-70% have Alzheimer's disease - the most common form of dementia - and with 10 million new cases each year, it has never been more important to equip ourselves with knowledge and understanding of this condition. If we are going to win the battle against dementia, then we need to help build dementia-friendly communities where people living with dementia are not stigmatised and stereotyped, and as a result mistreated, marginalised and isolated. If you are involved in the support of someone living with dementia, know someone with dementia or want to find out more about the condition, then this book offers exactly what you need. With no complicated jargon or medical terminology, it provides straightforward reading material to help you gain a good insight into what dementia is, what symptoms to look out for, and how to support someone living with dementia with a focus on the wellbeing of the person and not on the condition.

Glossary

Advocate a person responsible for acting and speaking on behalf of someone unable to do so.

Alzheimer's disease the most common type of dementia.

Assessment to carry out a formal or informal check and consider someone's abilities and symptoms, including strengths and weaknesses.

Dementia umbrella term used to describe the symptoms caused by diseases, syndromes, or damage to the brain that affect an individual's ability to think, remember, make decisions, or carry out daily living tasks.

Diagnosis identification of an illness by looking at the symptoms.

Duty of care a moral or legal obligation to ensure the wellbeing of others, keeping them safe from harm and neglect.

Empathy the ability to understand and share the feelings of another person.

Empower to enable someone to do something.

Hallucinations hear, see, smell, taste or feel things that appear to be real, but only exist in the mind.

Holistically as a whole, considering all aspects.

Mental capacity the ability to receive information, hold on to the information, weigh up the information, and make a decision based on the information.

Person-centred approach putting the person and his/her needs at the centre of the care and support we give him/her.

Personhood the quality or condition of being unique as an individual.

Power of Attorney the authority to act for another person in specific or all legal or financial matters.

Prevalence how often something occurs.

Risk factors the elements in someone's history or lifestyle that increase or decrease the chances of developing a specific condition.

Self- esteem how a person values him/herself.

Stereotype a generalised, fixed view of a particular type of person, group or thing.

Stereotyping making assumptions that all people in a particular group are the same.

Stigma a mark of disgrace or shame associated with a particular circumstance, quality, or person.

Symptoms physical or mental indicators of a condition or disease.

Vulnerable at greater risk of being harmed or affected, either physically or emotionally.

Meet Beulah

Beulah Shadrache is a specialist dementia consultant and researcher. With just under 20 years' experience in supporting people living with dementia and those involved in their care, Beulah has a passion for promoting their rights and helping improve systems to enhance their wellbeing and quality of life. As a health and social care lecturer and trainer Beulah is committed to empowering those involved in the lives and care of people living with dementia to ensure that they receive the best support. As a speaker, she takes bookings for speaking engagements, workshops, seminars and conferences.

Beulah is the founder of enABLE Foundation, a non-profit organisation dedicated to reducing the impact of dementia. Beulah can be contacted via the organisation's email address:

info@enablefoundation.org.